ESSENTIAL GUIDE TO BASAL CELL CARCINOMA

Comprehensive Insights and Treatment Strategies for the Most Common Skin Cancer

DR. CASEY LOREN

© 2024 by CASEY LOREN

All rights reserved .Except for brief quotations included in critical reviews and certain other noncommercial uses allowed by copyright law, no part of this book may be reproduced, distributed, or transmitted in any form or by any means, including photocopying, recording, or other electronic or mechanical methods, without the publisher's prior written permission.

DISCLAIMER

This book's content is only meant to be used for general informative purposes. Although the author has taken great care to ensure the content is accurate and thorough, no warranties or assurances on the information's accuracy, correctness, or reliability are provided. It is recommended that readers employ their own judgment and discretion when applying any material found in this book to their particular situation.

The information in this book is not intended to replace professional advice, nor is the author an expert in any of the subjects covered. It is recommended that readers consult with experienced professionals regarding any particular issues or concerns.

Any name that may be mentioned or referred in this book does not imply endorsement, recommendation, or relationship on the part of the author with any person, entity, good, website, or association. These references are made only for informational purposes and are not meant to be taken as recommendations or endorsements.

The information contained in this book may cause readers to suffer loss or damage, for which the author disclaims all obligation and accountability. The only people accountable for the decisions and actions taken by readers using the information presented are themselves.

Any names, characters, companies, locations, activities, occasions, and incidents referenced in this book are either made up or the result of the author's imagination. Any likeness to real people, living or dead, or to real things is entirely coincidental.

This book's content may change at any time, without prior notice, according to the author.

The onus is on the reader to verify whether there have been any updates or revisions.

The reader accepts the conditions of this disclaimer by reading this book. Please do not read this book or use its contents if you do not agree to these terms.

Table of Contents

CHAPTER 1

KNOWLEDGE OF BASAL CELL CARCINOMA

The lowest layer of the epidermis contains basal cells, which are the source of basal cell carcinoma (BCC), a kind of skin cancer. These cells are essential for the renewal and healing of the skin. BCC makes up almost 80% of all occurrences of skin cancer, making it the most prevalent kind.

Causes and Risk Factors:

The primary cause of BCC is ultraviolet (UV) light exposure from tanning beds or the sun.
Fair skin, a history of sunburns, a compromised immune system, exposure to specific chemicals, and a family history of skin cancer are additional risk factors.

Types of Cancer with Basal Cells:

BCC comes in a variety of subtypes, such as pigmented, morphea form, infiltrative, superficial, and nodular. Because each subtype is unique, it might need a different strategy for treatment.

Rates of Incidence and Prevalence:

BCC is very common, particularly in areas with lots of sun exposure. An estimated 4 million cases of BCC are diagnosed annually in the United States alone, while the disease's incidence rises throughout the world.

Symptoms and Indications:

Depending on the subtype, BCC can present with a variety of signs and symptoms, but they typically include a pearly or waxy bump, a flat, flesh-colored, or brown lesion that resembles a scar, a red or pink bump with a raised border and crusted center, or a sore that won't go away.

Methods of Diagnosis:

A comprehensive skin examination by a dermatologist, which may include a biopsy to confirm the presence of malignant cells as well as a visual inspection, is usually required for the diagnosis of BCC. In more advanced situations, imaging tests such as CT or ultrasound scans may be done to determine the cancer's extent.

The Value of Early Identification

A better prognosis and effective therapy depend on early identification of BCC. Better results and early diagnosis can be achieved by routine skin screenings, self-examinations, and quick review of any worrisome skin changes.

Assessment and Classification of Basal Cell Carcinoma:

Based on variables such as tumor size, invasion depth, involvement of surrounding structures, and metastatic presence, BCC is staged and graded. The staging process aids in choosing the best course of action and prognosis.

Rates of survival and prognosis:

When BCC is detected and treated early, the prognosis is usually quite good. For localized BCC, the five-year survival rate is around 100%; however, in situations of advanced or metastatic cancer, this rate may drop.

Effect on Life Quality:

Even though BCC is frequently curable, quality of life can still be significantly impacted by the diagnosis and course of treatment. Patients' well-being may be impacted by surgical procedures, scars, mental discomfort, and continuous surveillance, necessitating support from loved ones and medical professionals.

To encourage awareness, early detection, and efficient management of this prevalent form of skin cancer, patients, healthcare professionals, and the general public must have a thorough understanding of these characteristics of basal cell carcinoma.

CHAPTER 2
THE STRUCTURE AND FUNCTION OF THE SKIN

Skin's Structure:

The epidermis, dermis, and subcutaneous tissue make up the three primary layers of the skin, which is the biggest organ in the human body. The outermost layer, the epidermis, serves as a barrier to keep out viruses, UV rays, and environmental contaminants. Additionally, melanocytes are found there, generating melanin, the pigment that gives skin its color and shields it from UV rays. The dermis, which has blood vessels, nerves, sweat glands, and hair follicles, is located beneath the epidermis. The hypodermis, or subcutaneous tissue, is made up of fat cells that act as cushions and insulation.

Clinical Functions:

The skin carries out several crucial tasks that are necessary for general health. They include defense against pathogens, chemicals, and physical harm; control over body temperature through sweating and blood vessel dilation and constriction; perception of pressure, temperature, touch, and pain; production of vitamin D in response to sun exposure; and excretion of waste materials via sweat glands.

The epidermis' layers:

The stratum corneum, stratum lucidum, stratum granulosum, stratum spinosum, and stratum basale—also referred to as the stratum germinativum—are the layers that make up the epidermis. Every layer has unique properties and purposes. For example, the stratum basale is in charge of cell division and the synthesis of melanin, while the stratum corneum offers protection and waterproofing.

Subcutaneous Tissue and the Dermis:

Collagen and elastin fibers, which are abundant in the dermis, provide the skin its strength, suppleness, and support. It also contains nerves, sweat glands, sebaceous glands, blood arteries, and hair follicles. Adipose tissue, which acts as padding against external stresses, energy storage, and insulation, is found in the subcutaneous tissue.

Nails, Sweat Glands, and Hair:

The dermis contains hair follicles that create hair, which serves as protection and a sensory organ. Keratinized cells that make up nails shield fingertips and improve the perception of subtle touch. Sweat glands, which comprise both apocrine and eccrine glands, control body temperature and eliminate waste.

Melanocyte Role:

The pigment known as melanin, which gives skin its color, is produced by specialized cells called melanocytes in the epidermis. Melanin diffuses and absorbs UV radiation, protecting DNA from damage and lowering the risk of skin cancer.

Skin's Immune Function:

Through physical barriers, antimicrobial peptides, immune cells (including T lymphocytes and Langerhans cells), and cytokines, the skin plays a critical role in immunological defense. Together, these elements preserve skin homeostasis and offer protection against infections.

Skin Health Affected Factors:

Skin health is influenced by several factors, including age, hormone balance, nutrition, hydration, genetics, lifestyle choices (including drinking alcohol and smoking), exposure to pollutants and UV radiation from the environment, and skincare routines.

UV Radiation and Sun Exposure:

Sunlight's UV rays can harm skin cells, increasing the risk of skin cancers including basal cell carcinoma as well as sunburn and early aging. Minimising UV-related damage requires wearing protective clothing, using sunscreen, and finding shade during the hottest parts of the day.

In Development, Skin Cancer:

One type of skin cancer that commonly appears in areas exposed to UV radiation is basal cell carcinoma (BCC). It starts as a basal cell in the epidermis and might appear as a pink growth with elevated edges, a flat, flesh-colored, or brown scar-like lesion, or a pearly or waxy lump. To manage BCC and stop its progression, early detection and therapy are essential. Cryotherapy, topical treatments, Mohs micrographic surgery, and surgical excision are available treatment options. Skin cancer prevention and management require regular skin examinations, sun protection measures, and monitoring of skin changes.

CHAPTER 3

RISK ELEMENTS AND PREVENTIVE

Basal Cell Carcinoma Prevention Strategies and Risk Factors

UV Radiation and Sun Exposure:

The development of basal cell carcinoma (BCC) is closely linked to ultraviolet (UV) radiation exposure, mostly from the sun. The DNA in skin cells is harmed by prolonged and frequent exposure to UV radiation, which raises the possibility of developing BCC. Preventive measures include wearing long sleeves and hats, using broad-spectrum sunscreen frequently, and limiting sun exposure during peak hours.

Hereditary and Family Background:

Those who have a family history of BCC are more likely to get the illness. Genetic variables can affect how UV exposure affects skin cells. For those with a family history of BCC, routine tests and early detection are essential since they

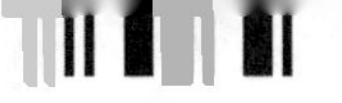

allow for the early implementation of preventive treatments.

Influence of Age and Gender:

Due to cumulative UV exposure over time, age is a significant risk factor for BCC, with older people being more vulnerable. When compared to women, men also experience a higher incidence of BCC. Understanding these demographic effects can help focus preventative initiatives, such as encouraging older men to wear sunscreen.

Complexion and Skin Type:

People with fair complexion, particularly those with light hair and eyes, are more likely to develop BCC. This is because their melanin levels are lower, which naturally protects against UV rays. Dermatologists' routine skin examinations and stringent sun protection measures are two preventative measures for this population.

Inhibition of immunity:

Individuals who have compromised immune systems, such as those who have received an organ transplant or suffer from specific medical problems, are more susceptible to acquiring BCC. The body's capacity to repair DNA damage from UV radiation can be hampered by immunosuppression. Strict adherence to sun protection measures and vigilant oversight by medical personnel are essential components of prevention.

Inhalation of Carcinogens:

BCC development may be facilitated by specific occupational exposures, such as those to radium, coal tar, or arsenic. Prevention requires reducing exposure to these carcinogens as much as possible through personal protective equipment and workplace safety procedures.

Prevention by Sunscreen Use:

Seeking shade, donning protective clothes, applying broad-spectrum sunscreen with an SPF of 30 or higher, and staying away from tanning beds are all good methods of preventing UV damage. The key to preventing BCC is educating people about these precautions and encouraging their regular adoption.

Survival Decisions for Prevention:

A balanced diet high in antioxidants, regular exercise, abstaining from tobacco and excessive alcohol use, and other healthy lifestyle choices can promote general skin health and lower the risk of BCC.

Value of Frequent Skin Examinations:

For the early detection of BCC, dermatologists or other healthcare professionals should regularly examine patients' skin. People must be urged to self-examine and report any changes in lesions, skin anomalies, or moles as soon as they occur.

Dermatologists' Function in Prevention:

Dermatologists are essential in the prevention of basal cell carcinoma (BCC) because they educate patients, screen for skin cancer, and create customized preventive programs based on individual risk factors. Additionally, they support public health campaigns that increase knowledge about early identification and prevention of skin cancer.

Through the management of these risk factors and the application of focused preventive techniques, people can greatly lower their chance of getting basal cell carcinoma and improve their skin health in general. To achieve this, regular cooperation between dermatologists, patients, and healthcare professionals is crucial.

CHAPTER 4

CAUSES AND PATHOPHYSIOLOGY OF BASAL CELL CARCINOMA

Genetic Mutations and Oncogenes: Genetic mutations and changes in oncogenes are frequently associated with basal cell carcinoma (BCC). In BCC cases, mutations in genes such as PTCH1, PTCH2, and SMO are frequently observed. These mutations cause unchecked cell proliferation and tumor formation by interfering with the regular operation of pathways involved in cell growth and differentiation.

UV Radiation Damage:

Exposure to ultraviolet (UV) radiation from artificial sources, such as tanning beds, or the sun is one of the main external causes that contributes to BCC. DNA damage is caused by UV radiation, especially to genes involved in DNA repair and cell cycle regulation. The likelihood of developing a BCC rises with time as a result of cumulative UV damage.

Immune System Dysfunction:

The pathogenesis of BCC may also be influenced by a weakened immune system. BCC is more likely to form in immunosuppressed people, such as those who have had organ transplants or certain autoimmune illnesses. Tumour growth results from aberrant cells being able to avoid identification and clearance due to a weaker immune response.

The Function of Tumour Suppressor Genes:

The preservation of cellular homeostasis and the inhibition of unchecked cell proliferation are made possible by tumor suppressor genes such as TP53 and PTEN. The development of BCC may be facilitated by mutations or inactivation of these genes, which may compromise their capacity to control apoptosis and cell division.

Inflammatory Pathways:

Another element linked to BCC is persistent inflammation. Through the creation of an environment that is favorable to cell proliferation and angiogenesis, inflammatory processes can aid in the beginning and advancement of tumors. In this situation, pro-inflammatory cytokines and signaling pathways are important.

Environmental Factors:

In addition to UV radiation, exposure to specific chemicals or poisons can raise the risk of breast cancer. For instance, exposure to arsenic has been connected to increased cases of bladder cancer, underscoring the significance of environmental regulation and monitoring.

Risk Factor Interaction:

The development of BCC can be influenced by the interaction of several risk factors, such as genetic predisposition, environmental exposures, and lifestyle variables like food and smoking. It is essential to comprehend these relationships to develop preventive measures and a thorough risk assessment.

Skin Microbiome Influence:

New research indicates that the development of BCC may be influenced by the skin microbiome, which is made up of a variety of microbial populations. The pathophysiology of BCC may be aided by dysbiosis or imbalance in the skin microbiota, which may affect immune responses and skin barrier functioning.

Emerging Research in Pathogenesis:

Current investigations are examining previously undiscovered facets of BCC pathogenesis, including the function of non-coding RNAs, epigenetic changes, and metabolic reprogramming in the development and spread of tumors. These discoveries may result in novel treatment targets and diagnostic markers.

Molecular Targets for therapy:

Thanks to developments in molecular biology, specific targets for BCC therapy have been found. Targeted medications that disrupt abnormal signaling pathways that promote tumor growth, such as hedgehog pathway inhibitors (vismodegib, sonidegib), have demonstrated effectiveness in treating advanced or recurring bladder cancer.

Comprehending the complex and multifaceted pathophysiology of BCC, encompassing immune system malfunction, UV exposure, genetic alterations, and environmental factors, is vital for formulating all-encompassing preventive and therapeutic approaches. Improving outcomes in BCC management may be possible by focusing on particular molecular pathways and incorporating new research discoveries.

CHAPTER 5
METHODS OF DIAGNOSIS AND SCREENING

Clinical Assessment

A comprehensive physical inspection of the patient's skin is part of the clinical examination, with special attention paid to any growths or lesions that seem suspicious. These tests are usually performed by dermatologists, who search for telltale signs such as uneven borders, telangiectasia (dilated blood vessels), pearly lumps, and ulceration.

Imaging and Dermoscopy

A dermatoscope, a portable device with light and magnification, is used in dermoscopy, a non-invasive procedure, to check skin lesions. It assists in distinguishing BCC from other skin disorders by assessing the structures within the lesion, such as pigment patterns and vascular systems. Diagnostic tools such as reflectance confocal microscopy (RCM), optical coherence tomography (OCT), and ultrasound can also produce fine-grained images of the skin's layers.

Skin Biopsy Techniques

A skin biopsy is frequently required for a conclusive BCC diagnosis. Depending on the size and location of the lesion, there are many biopsy procedures, such as punch, shave, and excisional biopsy. After that, a microscope examination of the biopsy sample is performed to determine the subtype and characteristics of BCC and to confirm its presence.

Pathological Examination

Histopathological analysis is the process of using a microscope to look at tissue samples from the biopsy to discover particular cellular characteristics of BCC. The tumor subtype (e.g., nodular, superficial, infiltrative), growth pattern, degree of differentiation, and the existence of any aggressive traits (e.g., perineural invasion) are all determined by this examination.

Chemical Analysis

Molecular testing can be used to identify genetic mutations linked to BCC, such as PTCH1 or TP53 gene alterations, using techniques like fluorescence in situ hybridization (FISH) or polymerase chain reaction (PCR). In situations of advanced or recurring BCC, in particular, these tests can assist guide treatment options by offering additional information regarding the molecular profile of the tumor.

Biomarkers and Blood Tests

Although blood tests are not commonly utilized for BCC diagnosis, they could be requested to evaluate general health and track any systemic consequences of advanced BCC. The potential role of biomarkers in predicting BCC risk, progression, and treatment response is also being investigated. Examples of these biomarkers include serum levels of specific proteins or enzymes.

Imaging investigations (MRI, PET-CT, CT)

In advanced cases of BCC, imaging studies such as computed tomography (CT), magnetic resonance imaging (MRI), and positron emission tomography-CT (PET-CT) are primarily used to assess for local invasion into surrounding structures or bones, detect any distant metastases, and determine the extent of tumor involvement.

Biopsy of the Sentinel Lymph Node

In certain cases with BCC, particularly when there is a suspicion of regional lymph node involvement, sentinel lymph node biopsy may be considered. To detect the sentinel lymph node and establish whether additional lymph node dissection is necessary, a tracer is injected close to the tumor site. The node is then excised and its contents are checked for cancerous cells.

Genetic Examination

Understanding the underlying genetic variables that contribute to the development of BCC involves genetic testing. It can detect genetic syndromes that are inherited and cause predispositions to numerous basal cell carcinomas and other tumors, such as Gorlin syndrome (nevoid basal cell carcinoma syndrome). In some circumstances, genetic testing and counseling may be advised, particularly for young individuals with numerous or early-onset BCCs.

Comprehensive Diagnostic Methodologies

To obtain a thorough evaluation of BCC, integrative diagnostic approaches integrate several methods, including clinical examination, dermoscopy, imaging, biopsy, and molecular testing. These methods seek to increase the precision of diagnoses, direct the choice of treatments, and efficiently track the advancement or recurrence of diseases.

Healthcare professionals can ensure prompt and accurate detection of basal cell carcinoma, resulting in appropriate management and better patient outcomes, by combining these many diagnostic and screening tools.

CHAPTER 6

OPTIONS FOR BASAL CELL CARCINOMA TREATMENT

Surgical Removal

Overview: To guarantee total removal, surgical excision entails removing the malignant tissue together with a margin of healthy tissue.

Advantages: It works well for the majority of BCCs, particularly the smaller or ones with well-defined borders. Pathological analysis verifies total elimination.

Thoughts: Might leave scars, and more substantial procedures might be needed for larger BCCs.

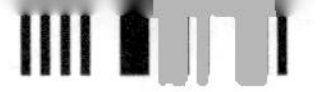

Micrographic Surgery with Mohs

Overview: Mohs surgery is a precise procedure in which tissue layers are cut away and then promptly checked under a microscope to ensure that no malignant cells are left.

Advantages: Excellent for regions with complex anatomy or recurrent BCCs, with high cure rates and little tissue damage.

Considerations: May need several stages, specific training and resources, and a significant investment of time.

Cryotherapy

Overview: Liquid nitrogen is used in cryotherapy to freeze and kill malignant tissue.

The technique is quick and outpatient, making it appropriate for superficial BCCs and leaving little scarring.

Considerations: Not appropriate for large or severe BCCs, less accurate than surgical techniques, and may need many treatments.

Electrodesiccation and Curettage

Overview: Curettage, the removal of malignant tissue, is followed by electrodesiccation, the use of an electric current to kill any remaining cells.

Advantages: Generally easy to do in an outpatient environment; good for superficial BCCs.

Considerations: May not be appropriate for some BCC kinds or sites; higher risk of recurrence in comparison to surgical excision or Mohs surgery.

Laser Treatment

Overview: Laser therapy targets and kills cancer cells with concentrated light.

Advantages: Accurate, little bleeding; in some situations, suitable for tiny, superficial BCCs.

Considerations: Limited penetration depth, not appropriate for all BCC kinds or locations, ongoing research is needed to gather long-term efficacy data.

Topical Pharmaceuticals

Overview: To treat superficial BCCs, the skin is treated with specific creams or gels (such as imiquimod and 5-fluorouracil).

Advantages: Non-invasive, appropriate for specific forms of BCC, patient-friendly.

Notes: Necessitates careful application, may irritate the skin, not appropriate for all BCCs (particularly those that are aggressive or profoundly invasive).

PDT stands for photodynamic therapy.

Overview: Photodynamic therapy (PDT) uses a photosensitizing chemical applied topically that is triggered by light to kill cancer cells.

Advantages: Non-invasive, appropriate for superficial BCCs, excellent cosmetic results.

Notes: Not appropriate for all BCC kinds; sensitivity to light after treatment; repeated sessions may be required.

Radiation Treatment

Overview: High-energy radiation is used in radiation treatment to kill cancer cells.

Advantages: Non-invasive, appropriate for regions where surgery presents difficulties, good aesthetic results for specific BCC subtypes.

Thoughts: Prolonged therapy, with possible adverse effects (e.g., alterations in skin tone, exhaustion), might not be appropriate for aggressive BCCs.

Specialised Treatments

Overview: Drugs known as targeted treatments, such as vismodegib and sonidegib, target particular pathways linked to the formation of BCCs.

Benefits: Oral medication in the form of pills for systemic treatment; effective for advanced or metastatic BCCs.

Thoughts: Pricey, not the first-line treatment for the majority of BCCs, potential side effects (such as muscular spasms and hair loss), etc.

Immunotherapy Choices

Overview: Immunotherapy medications, such as nivolumab and pembrolizumab, assist the immune system in identifying and eliminating cancer cells.

Advantages: Good for metastatic or advanced BCCs, systemic therapy, and potentially long-lasting effects.

Thoughts: Possible immunological adverse effects (rash, exhaustion, etc.), expensive, saved for particular situations.

Depending on the kind, location, size, and severity of the disease, each BCC treatment option has a role. The most qualified person to decide which course of action is best for a given patient is an oncologist or dermatologist.

CHAPTER 7

SURGICAL CARE AND RECONSTRUCTION

Procedure Scheduling

Surgery for basal cell carcinoma requires a thorough evaluation of the location, size, depth, and histological subtype of the tumor. It also takes into account the patient's past medical history, cosmetic issues, and general wellness. Whether using excision, Mohs surgery, or other procedures, the best surgical strategy is determined after a comprehensive inspection.

Margin and Extraction of Tumours

Selecting the right margins is essential to guarantee total excision of the malignant tissue while maintaining the integrity of the surrounding skin. The location and subtype of the tumor affect the margins. Clear margins are the goal of precise surgical methods, which lower the chance of recurrence.

Mohs Technique for Surgery

Mohs micrographic surgery is an extremely accurate method for removing BCCs, particularly when the tumors are located in places that are crucial to function or are aesthetically sensitive. To preserve healthy tissue as much as possible entails removing tissue layer by layer and immediately examining the sample under a microscope until no cancer cells are found.

Options for Reconstruction

Reconstruction after tumor excision aims to restore appearance and function. Primary closure, skin transplants, local flaps, and sophisticated methods such as tissue expansion or free flap reconstruction are among the options. The size, location, and patient-related considerations all influence the decision.

Procedures for Flaps

Following tumor removal, flap treatments entail transferring nearby tissue along with its blood supply to cover deficiencies. They produce outstanding functional and aesthetic results, especially for parts of the face with limited skin laxity or complex abnormalities.

Skin Grafting

To cover the surgical defect, skin grafting involves transferring healthy skin from a donor site. It is helpful for deep or big wounds for which flaps or primary closure are impractical. Grafts can be split-thickness or full-thickness, depending on the specifics of the lesion.

Considerations for Beautifying

A key component of BCC care is aesthetics, particularly when it comes to the face or other prominent places. During reconstruction, surgeons strive for symmetry, minimal scarring, and natural contours; frequently, they work in conjunction with plastic surgeons and dermatologists to maximize aesthetic results.

Scar Care

Scar management starts with careful closure procedures used during surgery. To enhance the appearance and texture of scars, postoperative treatments such as silicone gel sheets, corticosteroid injections, laser therapy, or scar revision operations may be suggested.

Aftercare

After BCC surgery, routine follow-up is crucial to track recovery, identify recurrence, and handle any issues right away. Clinical examinations, imaging scans, if necessary, and patient education on self-examination and sun protection are usually included in follow-up consultations.

Risk factors and complications

Although they are usually uncommon, BCC surgery complications can include nerve injury, hemorrhage, infection, poor wound healing, and unsatisfactory cosmetic results. Complication rates are influenced by risk factors such as tumor size, location, histological subtype, immunological condition of the patient, and prior treatments.

To get the best results, a complete approach to surgical management and reconstruction of basal cell carcinoma emphasizes the significance of customized techniques, multidisciplinary collaboration, and patient-centered care.

CHAPTER 8

NON-SURGICAL METHODS OF TREATMENT

Topic Treatments:

Medication administered topically is known as a topical therapy. They are usually applied to early-stage or superficial basal cell carcinomas. Topical therapies consist of diclofenac, imiquimod, and 5-fluorouracil (5-FU). These drugs either directly destroy malignant cells or activate the immune system to combat cancer. Because topical therapies are non-invasive, they are frequently chosen for tiny, low-risk lesions.

The use of liquid nitrogen and cryotherapy:

Through the use of liquid nitrogen, cancer cells are frozen during cryotherapy. This therapy is appropriate for basal cell carcinomas that are superficial. The lesion is directly treated with liquid nitrogen, which causes the cells to freeze and perish. It's a short process done in the doctor's office, and the treatment site may blister or cause some mild discomfort.

Laser Procedures:

High-energy light is used in laser therapy to kill cancer cells. For superficial or early-stage basal cell carcinomas, especially those on the face, it works well. With laser therapy, malignant cells can be precisely targeted with the least amount of harm to adjacent healthy tissue. Side effects are often minor and the recovery period is brief.

PDT, or photodynamic therapy:

PDT kills cancer cells by combining a medication called a photosensitizer with a particular kind of light. When treating superficial basal cell carcinomas, the photosensitizer is applied to the lesion, and it is subsequently exposed to light. PDT spares healthy tissue while targeting cancer cells specifically. Possible side effects include edema, redness, and transient photosensitivity.

Types of Radiation Therapy:

High-energy beams are used in radiation therapy to kill cancer cells. It is appropriate for basal cell carcinomas that are hard to treat surgically or in locations where surgery would not be possible, like the scalp or the vicinity of the eyes. Radiation therapy comes in two flavors: external beam radiation and brachytherapy, which involves applying radioactive material directly to the tumor or near it.

Medical Therapies Targeted:

Medication known as "targeted drug therapy" focuses on particular chemicals that contribute to the development of cancer. Examples are the inhibitors of the Hedgehog signaling system, vismodegib, and sonidegib, which are frequently mutated in basal cell cancer. These medications are used to treat metastatic or advanced basal cell carcinomas, and they have a great deal of success in slowing the growth of the tumor.

Agents for Immunotherapy:

Immunotherapy functions by inducing the immune system to identify and combat cancerous cells. When other treatments have failed to control advanced basal cell carcinomas, agents like pembrolizumab and nivolumab are utilized. Depending on the situation, immunotherapy can be employed as a first-line or supplementary treatment and has long-lasting effects.

Complementary Medicines:

Combination therapies aim to increase efficacy by utilizing two or more treatment methods either concurrently or consecutively. For instance, combining radiation therapy with topical therapies or immunotherapy with targeted medication therapy. Combination techniques are frequently customized to the needs of each patient and the properties of the tumor.

Conditioning Care:

Adjuvant therapies are extra medicines administered to lower the chance of a cancer recurrence following initial therapy. Depending on the circumstances, they could involve systemic drugs, radiation therapy, or topical treatments. Adjuvant therapies are intended to eradicate any cancer cells that may still be present and enhance long-term results.

Considering Palliative Care:

Enhancing the quality of life for patients with metastatic or advanced basal cell carcinoma is the main goal of palliative treatment. It deals with symptoms like weariness, pain, and emotional anguish. Palliative care teams collaborate with oncologists to offer all-encompassing treatment, which includes counseling, pain management, and help with end-of-life decisions.

Each of these non-surgical therapy modalities plays a key role in managing basal cell carcinoma, allowing patients alternatives tailored to their unique needs, tumor features, and stage of the disease.

CHAPTER 9

DEALING WITH CANCER OF THE BASAL CELL

Impact on Emotion

A person diagnosed with basal cell carcinoma (BCC) may experience a spectrum of feelings, including dread, anxiety, and sadness. It's critical to acknowledge and deal with these emotional effects:

- **Shock and Fear:** Many people feel shocked or incredulous when they receive a diagnosis. This is common, but it may be controlled by learning about BCC and the available treatments.

- **Anxiety and Uncertainty:** Anxiety might arise from the uncertainty of dealing with a cancer diagnosis. Having open lines of communication with support systems and medical professionals can help you handle these emotions.

- **Depression and Isolation:** Several people may feel depressed or alone. Emotional relief can be obtained by seeking assistance from support groups or mental health experts.

Coping Mechanisms

People with BCC can manage the difficulties of living using the following effective coping strategies:

- **Education:** Knowledge of BCC, available treatments, and prognosis can help people manage the condition more effectively.

- **Seeking assistance:** If you need emotional assistance, turn to friends, family, support groups, or mental health specialists.

- **Healthy Lifestyle:** Practices including regular exercise, a balanced diet, and enough sleep contribute to both physical and mental well-being.

- **Mindfulness and Relaxation Techniques:** Activities that promote relaxation and lower stress levels include deep breathing techniques, yoga, and meditation.

Assistance Mechanisms

Creating a solid support network is essential for adjusting to life with BCC:

- **Family and Friends:** Close ones can assist with everyday chores, accompany you to appointments, and offer emotional support.

- **Support Groups:** Participating in BCC-specific support groups enables people to meet others going through comparable struggles, exchange stories, and learn insightful things.

- **Healthcare Team:** Work collaboratively with medical specialists, such as dermatologists, counselors, and oncologists, to provide comprehensive support and treatment.

Modifications to Lifestyle

A few lifestyle adjustments can help control BCC and lower its risk factors:

- **Sun Protection:** Use sunscreen with a high SPF regularly and steer clear of prolonged sun exposure, especially during peak hours.

- **Stop Smoking:** Smoking raises the risk of cancer and exacerbates skin damage. Giving up smoking can lead to better general health results.

Healthy Diet: To promote the immune system and general health, eat a balanced diet high in fruits, vegetables, whole grains, and lean proteins.

Sun Safety Measures

It is imperative to engage in sun-safe practices to avoid BCC and reduce sun damage:

- **Use Sunscreen:** Every day, even on overcast days, use a broad-spectrum sunscreen with SPF 30 or higher.

- **Wear Protective clothes:** Use UV-protective clothes, caps, sunglasses, and long sleeves to cover exposed skin.

Seek Shade: Restrict your time in the sun, especially from 10 a.m. to noon. and 4:00 p.m. when the UV is at its strongest.

Routines for Skin Care

Developing a good skin care regimen can support healthy skin and the early identification of abnormalities:

- **Regular Skin Checks:** Examine yourself to keep an eye out for lesions, moles, and any changes to the texture or color of your skin. Inform medical professionals of any concerns as soon as possible.

- **Moisturise**: To keep skin hydrated and healthy, use moisturizers appropriate for your skin type.

- **Avoid strong Products:** Steer clear of strong chemicals or irritants that can harm your skin while using skincare products.

Succession Care Protocols

Monitoring the results of BCC treatment and identifying any recurrence or new lesions requires routine follow-up care:

- **Follow-Up Appointments:** Keep all agreed-upon follow-up appointments for skin examinations and assessments with medical professionals.

- **Imaging Tests:** Periodic imaging tests, such as CT scans, may be advised depending on the stage and course of treatment of the BCC.

- **Lifestyle Counselling:** During follow-up appointments, medical practitioners may provide advice on skincare, sun protection, and lifestyle changes.

Keeping an eye out for repeats

To find any indications of a BCC recurrence or new lesions, vigilant monitoring is essential:

- **Self-Exams:** Keep doing routine self-examinations to look for any changes in current lesions or growths.

Healthcare Provider Visits: Make follow-up appointments for comprehensive skin inspections and evaluations as directed by your healthcare providers.

- **Early Reporting:** Notify medical professionals right once of any unusual skin changes, including new growths, color or size changes, or bleeding.

Programmes for Survivorship

Following BCC treatment, survivorship programs provide persons with all-encompassing care and resources:

- **Education and Counselling:** Disseminate knowledge about healthy living after treatment, coping mechanisms, long-term effects, and surviving.

Support Services: Provide access to dietary counseling, mental health services, support groups, and rehabilitation initiatives.

Follow-Up Care Planning: Provide support in creating individualized plans for follow-up care, which may include monitoring schedules and lifestyle suggestions.

Awareness and Advocacy

The following are essential components of advocacy and awareness campaigns that support BCC prevention, early detection, and assistance:

- **Public Education:** Through public campaigns and educational activities, increase public knowledge of BCC risk factors, prevention options, and the significance of early detection.

Advocacy Groups: Support groups and advocacy groups devoted to policy advocacy, patient support, research, and awareness of skin cancer.

- **Community Engagement:** Promote sun-safe habits, skin cancer screenings, and support services by interacting with the neighborhood, healthcare providers, schools, and businesses.

Through a complete approach to these factors, people with Basal Cell Carcinoma can travel through their journey with increased self-assurance, empowerment, and support.

CHAPTER 10

RESEARCH DEVELOPMENTS AND UPCOMING PATHS

Present Directions in Basal Cell Carcinoma Research (BCC)

The present focus of research is to comprehend the underlying molecular mechanisms of BCC proliferation and development. Examining important signaling pathways like the Hedgehog pathway, which is essential to the pathophysiology of BCC, is one approach to do this. Finding unique genetic alterations linked to BCC and investigating the function of immune cells in the tumor microenvironment are two further trends.

New Treatment Targets for BCC, or basal cell carcinoma

Promising treatment targets for BCC have been found by recent research, including inhibitors of the Hedgehog pathway as vismodegib and sonidegib. Furthermore, in certain cases with advanced or metastatic BCC, immunotherapies that target immunological checkpoints such as PD-1 and PD-L1 have demonstrated success. Additionally being investigated are combination therapies that use immunotherapies in addition to targeted medicines.

Studies on Proteomics and Genomic Analysis in Basal Cell Carcinoma (BCC)

A better knowledge of the molecular profile of BCC has been attained by developments in genomic and proteomic research. These investigations have revealed particular genetic mutations and patterns of protein expression that are linked to the development of BCC and could be used as possible biomarkers for therapy response and diagnosis.

New Developments in Immunotherapy for Basal Cell Carcinoma (BCC)

Immunotherapy has become a viable treatment option for BCC, especially when other medicines are not working or should not be used. Adoptive cell therapy and immune checkpoint inhibitors are two tactics being researched, with good outcomes in terms of tumor reduction and extended survival in certain patients.

Development of Basal Cell Carcinoma (BCC) Biomarkers

Reliable biomarkers for BCC diagnosis, prognosis, and therapy response prediction are being developed. These biomarkers could come from immunohistochemical, proteomic, and genomic investigations; they could also include protein signatures, genetic markers, or immune cell profiles.

Artificial Intelligence in Basal Cell Carcinoma (BCC) Diagnostics

Enhancing the precision and effectiveness of tumor identification and classification is a major potential benefit of integrating artificial intelligence (AI) into BCC diagnosis. Dermatologists can receive assistance from AI algorithms that have been trained on extensive datasets in recognizing BCC lesions, differentiating them from other skin disorders, and forecasting their behavior.

Research with Patients at the Centre for Basal Cell Carcinoma (BCC)

Understanding each patient's particular requirements and preferences at every stage of their journey—from diagnosis to treatment and survivorship—is essential to a patient-centered approach to BCC research. This entails evaluating treatment satisfaction, psychosocial impact, quality of life, and participation in collaborative decision-making.

The landscape of basal cell carcinoma (BCC) clinical trials

The field of BCC clinical trials is changing quickly as new treatments, combination regimens, and biomarker-driven strategies are being studied. These trials seek to enhance results, lessen adverse effects, and customize treatment plans according to the unique needs of each patient.

Initiatives for Patient Education in Basal Cell Carcinoma (BCC)

Patient education programs are essential for enabling BCC patients to make knowledgeable decisions about their care. These programs encourage patient participation and adherence to advised recommendations by disseminating information about risk factors, early identification, treatment options, self-care techniques, and follow-up care.

Encouraging Advances in the Treatment of Basal Cell Carcinoma (BCC)

The introduction of targeted treatments, immunotherapies, and combination approaches—which provide better results and less toxicity than conventional medicines—are exciting advancements in the treatment of bladder cancer. Improvements in surgical methods, such as Mohs micrographic surgery, also help patients achieve improved functional and cosmetic results.

About improving the prognosis and standard of living for patients with basal cell carcinoma, each of these domains is essential to the field's clinical practice and research.

www.ingramcontent.com/pod-product-compliance
Lightning Source LLC
Chambersburg PA
CBHW061303250726
48653CB00002B/763